The Vibrant Lean & Green Cookbook

Easy Lean & Green Dishes For Weight Loss

Jesse Cohen

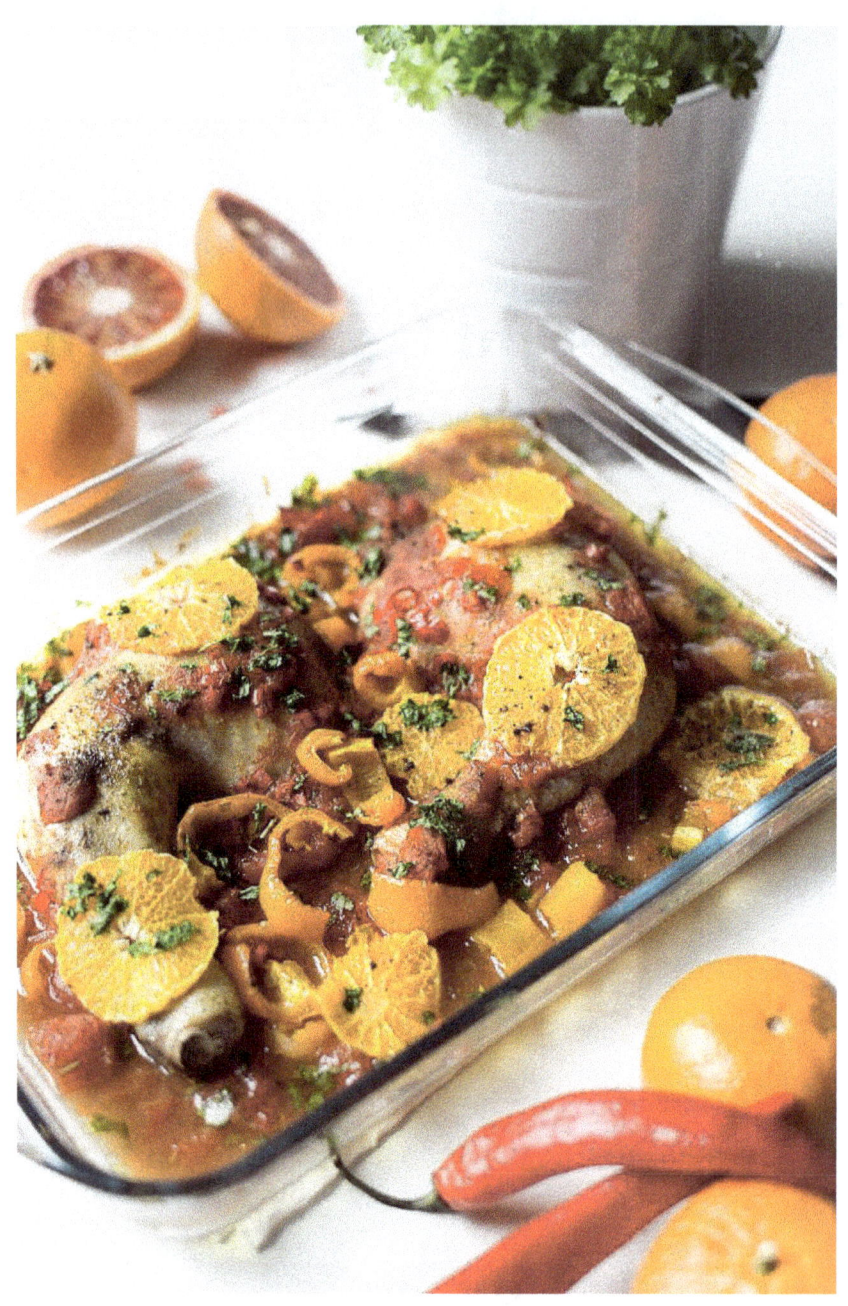

© Copyright 2020 - All rights reserved.

The content contained within this book may not be reproduced, duplicated or transmitted without direct written permission from the author or the publisher.

Under no circumstances will any blame or legal responsibility be held against the publisher, or author, for any damages, reparation, or monetary loss due to the information contained within this book. Either directly or indirectly.

Legal Notice:

This book is copyright protected. This book is only for personal use. You cannot amend, distribute, sell, use, quote or paraphrase any part, or the content within this book, without the consent of the author or publisher.

Disclaimer Notice:

Please note the information contained within this document is for educational and entertainment purposes only. All effort has been executed to present accurate, up to date, and reliable, complete information. No warranties of any kind are declared or implied. Readers acknowledge that the author is not engaging in the rendering of legal, financial, medical or professional advice. The content within this book has been derived from various sources. Please consult a licensed professional before attempting any techniques outlined in this book.

By reading this document, the reader agrees that under no circumstances is the author responsible for any losses, direct or indirect, which are incurred as a result of the use of information contained within this document, including, but not limited to, — errors, omissions, or inaccuracies.

Table of contents

Beef & Spinach Stew 7

Pork & Cabbage Stew 10

Salmon & Veggie Stew 12

Seafood & Spinach Stew 14

Herbed Seafood Stew 16

Spicy Chicken Legs 18

Marinated Chicken Legs 20

Gingered Chicken Drumsticks 22

Chicken Casserole 24

Instant Pot Chipotle Chicken & Cauliflower Rice Bowls 26

Tomato Cucumber Avocado Salad 28

Savory Cilantro Salmon 30

Chicken Zucchini Noodles 32

Lemon Garlic Oregano Chicken with Asparagus 35

Healthy Broccoli Salad 37

Parmesan Zucchini 39

Creamy Cauliflower Soup 42

Sheet Pan Chicken Fajita Lettuce Wraps 44

Taco Zucchini Boats 46

Salmon Florentine 49

Lean Pizza Hack 51

Amaranth Porridge 54

Lavender Blueberry Chia Seed Pudding 56

Coconut Chia Pudding with Berries 58

Omelette with Tomatoes and Spring Onions 60

Bacon Cheeseburger 62

Chia Seed Gel with Pomegranate and Nuts 65

Pancakes with Berries 67

Porridge with Walnuts 70

Omelette à la Margherita 72

Sweet Cashew Cheese Spread 74

Personal Biscuit Pizza 76

Fried Egg with Bacon 78

Eel on Scrambled Eggs and Bread 80

Whole Grain Bread and Avocado 82

Cheeseburger Pie 84

Asparagus & Crabmeat Frittata 86

Grilled Chicken Power Bowl with Green Goddess Dressing 88

Yogurt with Granola and Persimmon 91

Smoothie Bowl with Spinach, Mango, and Muesli 93

Smoothie Bowl with Berries, Poppy Seeds, Nuts and Seeds 95

Mini Zucchini Bites 97

Beef with Broccoli on Cauliflower Rice 99

Ancho Tilapia on Cauliflower Rice 101

Turkey Caprese Meatloaf Cups 103

Almond Pancakes 105

Beef & Spinach Stew

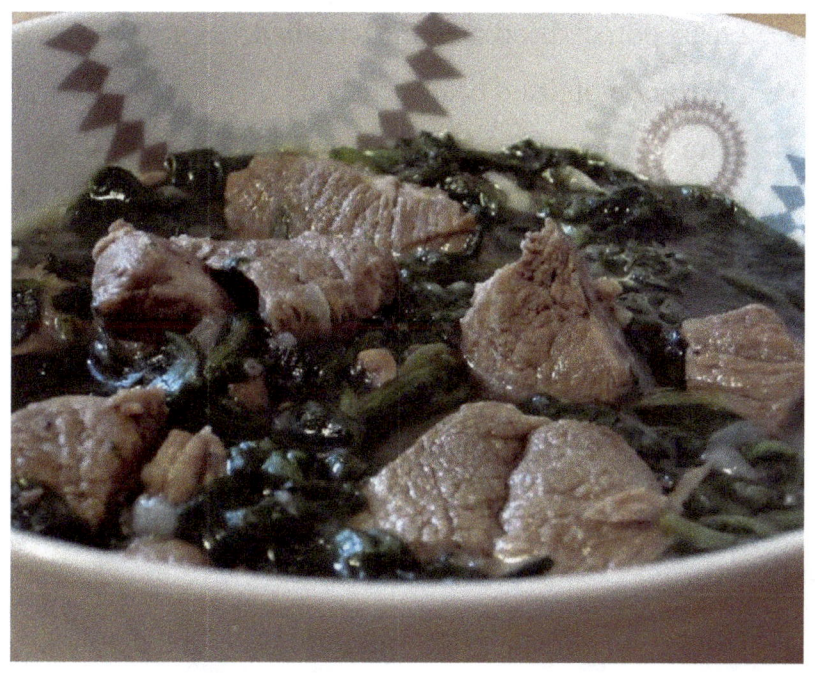

Servings: 10

Preparation Time: 15 minutes

Cooking Time: 6 hours 10 minutes

Ingredients:

- ¼ cup of olive oil, divided
- 2½ pounds beef stew meat, cubed
- Salt and ground black pepper, as required

- 2 small onions, chopped
- 1 teaspoon of dried thyme, crushed
- 1 teaspoon of dried oregano, crushed
- 1 teaspoon of dried basil, crushed
- 1 cup of carrot, peeled and chopped
- 1 celery stalk, chopped
- 10 cups of fresh spinach, chopped
- 1 cup of fresh tomatoes, chopped finely
- 2 cups of chicken broth
- 3 tablespoons of fresh lemon juice

Instructions:

1. In an oven-safe pan that will put in the Breville Smart Air Fryer Oven, heat 2 tablespoons of the oil over medium heat and cook the meat cubes with salt and black pepper for about 4-5 minutes.
2. With a slotted spoon, transfer the meat cubes into a bowl.
3. In the pan, add the remaining oil and onions and cook for about 4-5 minutes.
4. Remove from the heat and stir in the cooked beef and remaining ingredients apart from lemon juice.
5. Cover the pan with a lid.
6. Arrange the pan over the wire rack.

7. Select "Slow Cooker" of Breville Smart Air Fryer Oven and assail "Low".
8. Set the timer for six hours and press "Start/Stop" to start cooking.
9. When the cooking time is completed, remove the pan from the oven and serve hot.
10. Open the lid and stir in the lemon juice.
11. Serve hot.

Pork & Cabbage Stew

Servings: 8

Preparation Time: 15 minutes

Cooking Time: 7½ hours

Ingredients:

- 2½ pounds boneless pork meat, cubed into 2-inch size
- 2½ cups of cabbage, chopped
- 2 cups of tomatoes, chopped finely
- 1 medium onion, chopped
- 2 garlic cloves, minced
- 2 tablespoons of olive oil
- 4 cups of chicken broth
- 1 tablespoon of fresh oregano, minced
- Salt and ground black pepper, as required
- 3 tablespoons of fresh lime juice

Instructions:

1. In an oven-safe pan that will put in the Breville Smart Air Fryer Oven, place all ingredients and stir to mix.
2. Cover the pan with a lid.
3. Arrange the pan over the wire rack.

4. Select "Slow Cooker" of Breville Smart Air Fryer Oven and assail "Low".
5. Set the timer for 7½ hours and press "Start/Stop" to start cooking.
6. When the cooking time is completed, remove the pan from the oven and serve hot.
7. Open the lid and transfer pork into a large bowl.
8. With 2 forks, shred the meat.
9. Return the shredded pork into the pan and blend well.
10. Serve hot with the drizzling of lemon juice.

Salmon & Veggie Stew

Servings: 4

Preparation Time: 15 minutes

Cooking Time: 6 hours

Ingredients:

- 1-pound salmon fillet, cubed
- 1 tablespoon of coconut oil
- 1 medium yellow onion, chopped
- 1 garlic clove, minced
- 1 zucchini, sliced
- 1 green bell pepper, seeded and cubed
- ½ cup of tomatoes, chopped
- ½ cup of fish broth
- ¼ teaspoon of dried oregano
- ¼ teaspoon of dried basil
- Salt and ground black pepper, as required

Instructions:

1. In an oven-safe pan that will put in the Breville Smart Air Fryer Oven, place all ingredients and stir to mix.
2. Cover the pan with a lid.

3. Arrange the pan over the wire rack.
4. Select "Slow Cooker" of Breville Smart Air Fryer Oven and assail "Low".
5. Set the timer for 5-6 hours and press "Start/Stop" to start cooking.
6. When the cooking time is completed, remove the pan from the oven and serve hot.

Seafood & Spinach Stew

Servings: 8

Preparation Time: 20 minutes

Cooking Time: 4 hours 50 minutes

Ingredients:

- 2 tablespoons of olive oil
- ½ pound tomatoes, chopped
- 1 large yellow onion, chopped finely
- 2 garlic cloves, minced
- 2 teaspoons of curry powder
- 6 sprigs fresh parsley
- Salt and ground black pepper, as required
- 1½ cups of chicken broth
- 1½ pounds salmon, cut into cubes
- 1½ pounds shrimp, peeled and deveined
- 1-pound fresh spinach, chopped

Instructions:

1. In an oven-safe pan that will put in the Breville Smart Air Fryer Oven, place all ingredients apart from seafood and spinach and stir to mix.

2. Cover the pan with a lid.
3. Arrange the pan over the wire rack.
4. Select "Slow Cooker" of Breville Smart Air Fryer Oven and assail "Low".
5. Set the timer for 4 hours and press "Start/Stop" to start cooking.
6. When the cooking time is completed, remove the pan from the oven.
7. Open the lid and stir in the seafood and spinach.
8. Cover the pan with a lid.
9. Arrange the pan over the wire rack.
10. Select "Slow Cooker" of Breville Smart Air Fryer Oven and assail "Low".
11. Set the timer for 50 minutes and press "Start/Stop" to start cooking.
12. When the cooking time is completed, remove the pan from the oven and serve hot.

Herbed Seafood Stew

Servings: 8

Preparation Time: 20 minutes

Cooking Time: 4¾ hours

Ingredients:

- 1 small celery stalk, chopped
- 1 small carrot, peeled and chopped
- 1 yellow onion, chopped
- 3 garlic cloves, chopped
- 1 cup of fresh cilantro leaves, chopped
- 1 cup of tomatoes, chopped finely
- 4 cups of chicken broth
- 2 tablespoons of fresh lemon juice
- 2 tablespoons of olive oil
- 3 teaspoons of mixed dried herbs (rosemary, thyme, marjoram)
- Salt and ground black pepper, as required
- 1-pound cod fillets, cubed
- 1-pound shrimp, peeled and deveined
- 1-pound scallops
- ¾ cup of crabmeat

Instructions:

1. In an oven-safe pan that will put in the Breville Smart Air Fryer Oven, place all ingredients apart from seafood and stir to mix.
2. Cover the pan with a lid.
3. Arrange the pan over the wire rack.
4. Select "Slow Cooker" of Breville Smart Air Fryer Oven and assail "Low".
5. Set the timer for 4 hours and press "Start/Stop" to start cooking.
6. When the cooking time is completed, remove the pan from the oven.
7. Open the lid and stir in the seafood.
8. Cover the pan with a lid.
9. Arrange the pan over the wire rack.
10. Select "Slow Cooker" of Breville Smart Air Fryer Oven and assail "Low".
11. Set the timer for 45 minutes and press "Start/Stop" to start cooking.
12. When the cooking time is completed, remove the pan from the oven and stir the mixture well.
13. Serve hot.

Spicy Chicken Legs

Servings: 6

Preparation Time: 15 minutes

Cooking Time: 25 minutes

Ingredients:

- 2½ pounds of chicken legs
- 2 tablespoons of olive oil
- 1 teaspoon of smoked paprika
- 1 teaspoon of garlic powder
- ½ teaspoon of ground cumin
- Salt and ground black pepper, as required
- 8 cups of fresh baby greens

Instructions:

1. In a large bowl, add all the ingredients apart from baby greens and blend well.
2. Arrange the chicken legs onto the greased enamel roasting pan.
3. Select "Air Fry" of Breville Smart Air Fryer Oven and adjust the temperature to 400 degrees F.

4. Set the timer for 25 minutes and press "Start/Stop" to start preheating.
5. When the unit beeps to point out that it's preheated, insert the roasting pan in the oven.
6. When the cooking time is completed, remove the roasting pan from the oven and transfer the chicken pieces onto a platter.
7. Serve hot alongside the baby greens.

Marinated Chicken Legs

Servings: 4

Preparation Time: 15 minutes

Cooking Time: 20 minutes

Ingredients:

- 4 chicken legs
- 3 tablespoons of fresh lemon juice
- 3 teaspoons of ginger paste
- 3 teaspoons of garlic paste
- Salt, as required
- 4 tablespoons of low-fat plain yogurt
- 2 teaspoons of red chili powder
- 1 teaspoon of ground cumin
- 1 teaspoon of ground coriander
- 1 teaspoon of ground turmeric
- Ground black pepper, as required
- 6 cups of fresh baby kale

Instructions:

1. In a bowl, chicken legs, lemon juice, ginger paste, garlic paste, and salt and blend well.

2. Put aside for about 15 minutes.
3. Meanwhile, in another bowl, mix the yogurt, spices, and coloring.
4. Add the chicken legs into the bowl and generously coat with the spice mixture.
5. Cover the bowl of chicken and refrigerate for at least 10-12 hours.
6. Arrange the chicken legs into the greased air fry basket.
7. Select "Air Fry" of Breville Smart Air Fryer Oven and adjust the temperature to 445 degrees F.
8. Set the timer for 20 minutes and press "Start/Stop" to start preheating.
9. When the unit beeps to point out that it's preheated, insert the air fry basket in the oven.
10. When the cooking time is completed, remove the air fry basket from the oven and serve hot alongside the kale.

Gingered Chicken Drumsticks

Servings: 3

Preparation Time: 10 minutes

Cooking Time: 25 minutes

Ingredients:

For Drumsticks:

- ¼ cup of full-fat coconut milk
- 2 teaspoons of fresh ginger, minced
- 2 teaspoons of galangal, minced
- 2 teaspoons of ground turmeric
- Salt, as required
- 3 (6-ounce of) chicken drumsticks

For Serving:

- 6 cups of fresh spinach

Instructions:

1. In a large bowl, add the coconut milk, galangal, ginger, and spices and blend well.
2. Add the chicken drumsticks and coat with the marinade generously.

3. Refrigerate to marinate for at least 6-8 hours.
4. Arrange the chicken drumsticks onto the greased enamel roasting pan.
5. Select "Air Fry" of Breville Smart Air Fryer Oven and adjust the temperature to 375 degrees F.
6. Set the timer for 25 minutes and press "Start/Stop" to start preheating.
7. When the unit beeps to point out that it's preheated, insert the roasting pan in the oven.
8. When the cooking time is completed, remove the roasting pan from the oven and transfer the chicken drumsticks onto plates.
9. Serve hot alongside the spinach.

Chicken Casserole

Preparation Time: 15 minutes

Cooking Time: 40 minutes

Servings: 4

Ingredients:

- 1 lb. of cooked chicken; shredded
- ¼ cup of Greek yogurt
- 1 cup of cheddar cheese; shredded
- ½ cup of salsa
- 4 oz. of cream cheese; softened
- 4 cups of cauliflower florets
- 1/8 tsp. of black pepper
- ½ tsp. of kosher salt

Directions:

1. Add cauliflower florets into the microwave-safe dish and cook for 10 minutes or until soft.
2. Add cheese and microwave for 30 seconds more. Stir well.

3. Add chicken, yogurt, cheddar cheese, salsa, pepper, and salt and stir everything well.
4. Preheat the oven to 375° F.
5. Bake in preheated oven for 20 minutes.
6. Serve hot and enjoy.

Nutrition:
- Calories: 429
- Fat: 23 g
- Carbs: 6 g
- Sugar: 7 g
- Protein: 44 g
- Cholesterol: 149 mg

Instant Pot Chipotle Chicken & Cauliflower Rice Bowls

Preparation Time: 10 minutes

Cooking Time: 20 minutes

Servings: 4

Ingredients:

- 1/3 cup of salsa
- 1 quantity of 14.5 oz. of can fire-roasted diced tomatoes
- 1 canned chipotle pepper + 1 teaspoon sauce
- ½ teaspoon of dried oregano
- 1 teaspoon of cumin
- 1 ½ lb. of boneless, skinless chicken breast
- ¼ teaspoon of salt
- 1 cup of reduced-fat shredded Mexican cheese blend
- 4 cups of frozen diced cauliflower
- ½ medium-sized avocado, sliced

Directions:

1. Combine the primary ingredients in a blender and blend until they become smooth.
2. Place the chicken in its pot and pour the sauce over it. Cover the lid and shut the pressure valve. Put it on high heat for 20 minutes. Allow the pressure release on its own before opening. Remove the chicken, and then add it back to the sauce.
3. Microwave the diced cauliflower according to the directions on the package.
4. Before you serve, divide the diced cauliflower, cheese, avocado, and chicken equally among the 4 bowls.

Nutrition:

- Calories: 287
- Protein: 35 g
- Carbohydrate: 19 g
- Fat: 12 g

Tomato Cucumber Avocado Salad

Preparation Time: 15 minutes

Cooking Time: 0 minutes

Servings: 4

Ingredients:

- 12 oz. of cherry tomatoes, cut in half
- 5 small cucumbers; chopped
- 3 small avocados; chopped
- ½ tsp. of ground black pepper
- 2 tbsps. of olive oil
- 2 tbsps. of fresh lemon juice
- ¼ cup of fresh cilantro; chopped
- 1 tsp. of sea salt

Directions:

1. Add cherry tomatoes, cucumbers, avocados, and cilantro into the massive bowl and blend well.
2. Mix olive oil, lime juice, black pepper, and salt together and pour over the salad.

3. Toss well and serve immediately.

Nutrition:
- Calories: 442
- Fat: 31 g
- Carbs: 30.3 g
- Sugar: 4 g
- Protein: 2 g
- Cholesterol: 0 mg

Savory Cilantro Salmon

Preparation Time: 10 minutes

Cooking Time: 30 minutes

Servings: 4

Ingredients:

- 2 tablespoons of fresh lime or lemon
- 4 cups of fresh cilantro; divided
- 2 tablespoon of hot red pepper sauce
- ½ teaspoon of salt; divided
- 1 teaspoon of cumin
- 4, 7 oz. of salmon filets
- ½ cup of (4 oz.) water
- 2 cups of sliced red bell pepper
- 2 cups of sliced yellow bell pepper
- 2 cups of sliced green bell pepper
- Cooking spray
- ½ teaspoon of pepper

Directions:

1. Get a blender or food processor and mix half the cilantro, juice or lemon, cumin, hot red Poivrade, water, and salt; then puree until they become smooth. Transfer the marinade gotten into a large re-sealable bag.
2. Add salmon to marinade. Seal the bag, squeeze out air which may be trapped inside, add coat salmon. Refrigerate for about 1 hour, turning as often as possible.
3. Now, after marinating, preheat your oven to about 400° F. Arrange the pepper slices in a single layer in a slightly greased, medium-sized square baking dish. Bake it for 20 minutes, then turn the pepper slices once.
4. Drain your salmon and do away with the marinade. Crust the upper part of the salmon with the remaining chopped, fresh cilantro. Place salmon on the top of the pepper slices and bake for about 12-14 minutes or until you notice that the fish flakes easily when it is tested with a fork. Enjoy.

Nutrition:

Calories: 350

Carbohydrate: 15 g

Protein: 42 g

Fat: 13 g

Chicken Zucchini Noodles

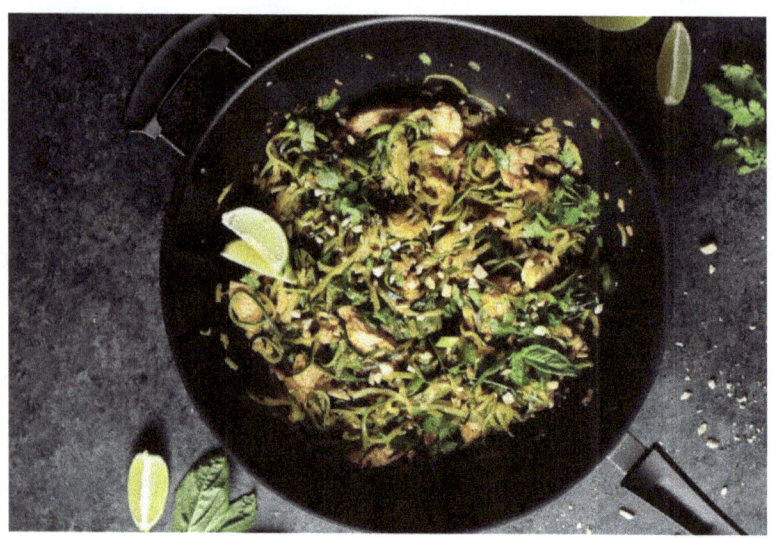

Preparation Time: 20 minutes

Cooking Time: 5 minutes

Servings: 2

Ingredients:

- 1 large zucchini, spiralized
- 1 chicken breast; skinless & boneless
- ½ tbsp. of jalapeno; minced
- 2 garlic cloves, minced
- ½ tsp. of ginger; minced

- ½ tbsp. fish sauce
- 2 tbsps. of coconut cream
- ½ tbsp. of honey
- ½ lime juice
- 1 tbsp. of peanut butter
- 1 carrot, chopped
- 2 tbsps. of cashews; chopped
- ¼ cup of fresh cilantro; chopped
- 1 tbsp. of olive oil
- Pepper
- Salt

Directions:
1. Heat vegetable oil in a pan over medium-high heat.
2. Season chicken breast with pepper and salt. Once the oil is hot then add chicken breast into the pan and cook for 3-4 minutes per side or until properly cooked.
3. Remove chicken breast from pan. Shred chicken breast with a fork and put aside.
4. In a small bowl, mix jalapeno, garlic, ginger, fish sauce, coconut milk, honey, and juice together. Set aside.

5. In a large bowl, combine together spiralized zucchini, carrots, cashews, cilantro, and shredded chicken.
6. Pour spread mixture over zucchini noodles and toss to mix.
7. Serve immediately and enjoy.

Nutrition:

- Calories 353
- Fat: 21 g
- Carbs: 20.5 g
- Sugar: 8 g
- Protein: 25 g
- Cholesterol: 54 mg

Lemon Garlic Oregano Chicken with Asparagus

Preparation Time: 5 minutes

Cooking Time: 40 minutes

Servings: 4

Ingredients:

- 1 small lemon, juiced (this should be about 2 tablespoons of lemon juice)
- 1 ¾ lb. of bone-in, skinless chicken thighs
- 2 tablespoon of fresh oregano, minced
- 2 cloves of garlic; minced
- 2 lbs. of asparagus; trimmed
- ¼ teaspoon each or less for black pepper and salt

Directions:

1. Preheat the oven to about 350º F.
2. Put the chicken in a medium-sized bowl. Now, add the garlic, oregano, lemon juice, pepper, and salt and toss together to mix.

3. Roast the chicken in the air fryer oven until it reaches an indoor temperature of 165º F in about 40 minutes. Once the chicken thighs are cooked, remove and keep aside to rest.
4. Now, steam the asparagus on a stovetop or in a microwave to the specified doneness.
5. Serve asparagus with the roasted chicken thighs.

Nutrition:

- Calories: 350
- Fat: 10 g
- Carbohydrate: 10 g
- Protein: 32 g

Healthy Broccoli Salad

Preparation Time: 25 minutes

Cooking Time: 0 minutes

Servings: 6

Ingredients:

- 3 cups of broccoli; chopped
- 1 tbsp. of apple cider vinegar
- ½ cup of Greek yogurt
- 2 tbsps. of sunflower seeds
- 3 bacon slices; cooked and chopped
- 1/3 cup of onion; sliced
- ¼ tsp. of stevia

Directions:

1. In a bowl, mix together broccoli, onion, and bacon.
2. In a small bowl, mix together yogurt, vinegar, stevia, and pour over the broccoli mixture. Stir to mix.
3. Sprinkle sunflower seeds on top of the salad.
4. Store salad in the refrigerator for 30 minutes.

5. Serve and enjoy.

Nutrition:

- Calories 90
- Fat: 9 g
- Carbs: 4 g
- Sugar: 5 g
- Protein: 2 g
- Cholesterol: 12 mg

Parmesan Zucchini

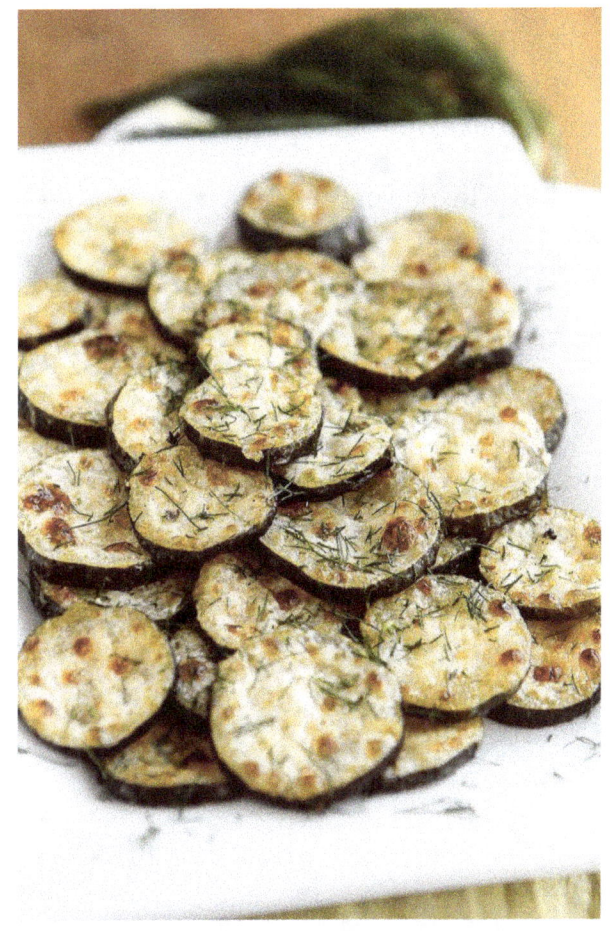

Preparation Time: 15 minutes

Cooking Time: 15 minutes

Servings: 4

Ingredients:

- 4 zucchini; quartered lengthwise
- 2 tbsp. of fresh parsley; chopped
- 2 tbsps. of olive oil
- ¼ tsp. of garlic powder
- ½ tsp. of dried basil
- ½ tsp. of dried oregano
- ½ tsp. of dried thyme
- ½ cup of parmesan cheese; grated
- Pepper
- Salt

Directions:

1. Preheat the oven to 350° F. Line baking sheet with parchment paper and put aside.
2. In a small bowl, mix together parmesan cheese, garlic powder, basil, oregano, thyme, pepper, and salt.
3. Arrange zucchini on the prepared baking sheet, drizzle with oil and sprinkle with parmesan cheese mixture.

4. Bake in preheated oven for 15 minutes then broil for 2 minutes or until lightly golden brown.
5. Garnish with parsley and serve immediately.

Nutrition:

- Calories: 244
- Fat: 14 g
- Carbs: 7 g
- Sugar: 5 g
- Protein: 15 g
- Cholesterol: 30 mg

Creamy Cauliflower Soup

Preparation Time: 15 minutes

Cooking Time: 15 minutes

Servings: 6

Ingredients:

- 5 cups of cauliflower rice
- 8 oz. of cheddar cheese; grated
- 2 cups of unsweetened almond milk
- 2 cups of vegetable stock
- 2 tbsps. of water
- 1 small onion; chopped
- 2 garlic cloves; minced
- 1 tbsp. of olive oil
- Pepper
- Salt

Directions:

1. Heat olive oil in a large stockpot over medium heat.

2. Add onion and garlic and cook for 1-2 minutes.
3. Add cauliflower rice and water. Cover and cook for 5-7 minutes.
4. Now add vegetable stock and almond milk and stir well. Bring to a boil.
5. Turn heat to low and simmer for five minutes.
6. Turn off the heat. Slowly add cheddar and stir until smooth.
7. Season soup with pepper and salt.
8. Stir well and serve hot.

Nutrition:

- Calories: 214
- Fat: 15 g
- Carbs: 3 g
- Sugar: 3 g
- Protein: 16 g
- Cholesterol: 40 mg

Sheet Pan Chicken Fajita Lettuce Wraps

Preparation Time: 15 minutes

Cooking Time: 30 minutes

Servings: 2

Ingredients:

- 1 lb. of chicken breast; thinly sliced into strips
- 2 teaspoons of olive oil
- 2 bell peppers; thinly sliced into strips
- 2 teaspoons of fajita seasoning
- 6 leaves from a romaine heart
- Juice of half a lime
- ¼ cup of plain of non-fat Greek yogurt

Directions:

1. Preheat your oven to about 400° F.
2. Combine all of the ingredients apart from lettuce in a large bag which will be resealed. Mix alright to coat vegetables and chicken with oil and seasoning evenly.

3. Spread the contents of the bag evenly on a foil-lined baking sheet. Bake it for about 25-30 minutes, or until the chicken is thoroughly cooked.
4. Serve on lettuce leaves and top with Greek yogurt if you wish.

Nutrition:

- Calories: 387
- Fat: 6 g
- Carbohydrate: 14 g
- Protein: 18 g

Taco Zucchini Boats

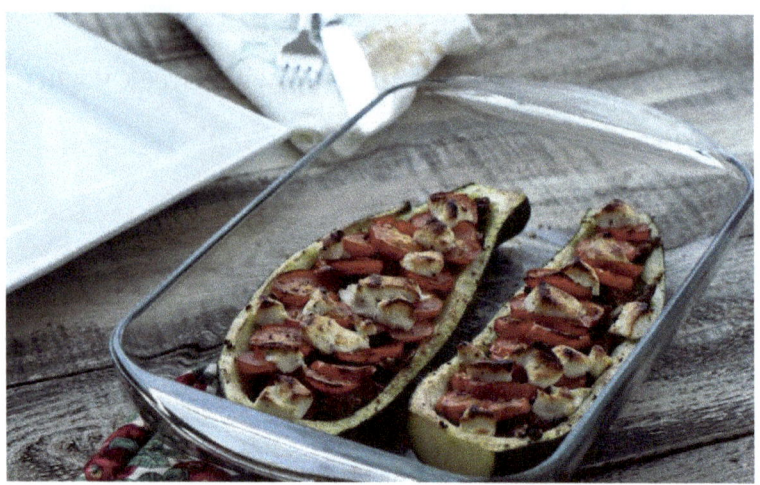

Preparation Time: 20 minutes

Cooking Time: 55 minutes

Servings: 4

Ingredients:

- 4 medium zucchinis; cut in half lengthwise
- ¼ cup of fresh cilantro; chopped
- ½ cup of cheddar cheese; shredded
- ¼ cup of water
- 4 oz. of tomato sauce

- 2 tbsps. of bell pepper; minced
- ½ small onion; minced
- ½ tsp. of oregano
- 1 tsp. of paprika
- 1 tsp. of chili powder
- 1 tsp. of cumin
- 1 tsp. of garlic powder
- 1 lb. of lean ground turkey
- ½ cup of salsa
- 1 tsp. of kosher salt

Directions:
1. Preheat the oven to 400º F.
2. Add ¼ cup of salsa at the bottom of the baking dish.
3. Use a spoon to hollow the middle of the zucchini halves.
4. Chop the scooped-out flesh of zucchini and put aside ¾ of a cup chopped flesh.
5. Add zucchini halves in the boiling water and cook for 1 minute. Remove zucchini halves from water.
6. Add ground turkey in a large pan and cook until meat is no longer pink. Add spices and blend well.

7. Add the remaining zucchini halves, water, spaghetti sauce, bell pepper, and onion. Stir well and cover, then simmer over low heat for 20 minutes.
8. Stuff zucchini boats with taco meat and top each with one tablespoon of shredded cheddar.
9. Place zucchini boats in baking dish. Cover dish with foil and bake in preheated oven for 35 minutes.
10. Top with remaining salsa and chopped cilantro.
11. Serve and enjoy.

Nutrition:

- Calories: 297
- Fat: 17 g
- Carbs: 12 g
- Sugar: 3 g
- Protein: 30.2 g
- Cholesterol: 96 mg

Salmon Florentine

Preparation Time: 5 minutes

Cooking Time: 30 minutes

Servings: 4

Ingredients:

- 1 ½ cups of chopped cherry tomatoes
- ½ cup of chopped green onions
- 2 garlic cloves; minced
- 1 teaspoon of olive oil
- 1, 12 oz. package frozen chopped spinach; thawed and patted dry
- ¼ teaspoon of crushed red pepper flakes
- ½ cup of part-skim ricotta cheese
- ¼ teaspoon each for pepper and salt
- 4, 5 ½ oz. wild salmon fillets
- Cooking spray

Directions:

1. Preheat the oven to 350° F.
2. Use a medium skillet to cook onions in oil until they start to melt, which should be in about 2 minutes. You can then add garlic inside the skillet and cook for an additional 1 minute. Add the spinach, red pepper flakes, tomatoes, pepper, and salt. Cook for 2 minutes while stirring. Remove the pan from the heat and let it cool for about 10 minutes. Stir in the ricotta.
3. Put 1/4 of the spinach mixture on top of every salmon fillet. Place the fillets on a slightly-greased rimmed baking sheet and bake it for 15 minutes or until you are sure that the salmon has been thoroughly cooked.

Nutrition:

- Calories: 350
- Carbohydrate: 15 g
- Protein: 42 g
- Fat: 13 g

Lean Pizza Hack

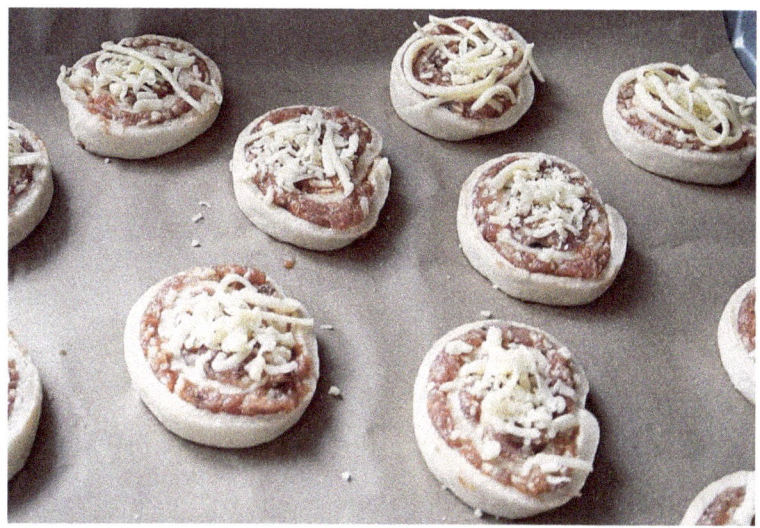

Preparation Time: 5-10 minutes

Cooking Time: 15-20 minutes

Servings: 1

Ingredients:

- 1/4 fueling of garlic mashed potato
- 1/2 egg whites
- 1/4 tablespoon of baking powder
- 3/4 oz. of reduced-fat shredded mozzarella
- 1/8 cup of sliced white mushrooms

- 1/16 cup of pizza sauce
- 3/4 oz. of ground beef
- 1/4 sliced black olives
- You also need a sauté pan, baking sheets, and parchment paper

Directions:

1. Start by preheating the oven to 400°F.
2. Mix your baking powder and garlic potato packet.
3. Add egg whites to your mixture and stir well until it blends.
4. Line the baking sheet with parchment paper and pour the mixed batter onto it.
5. Put another parchment paper on top of the batter and open up the batter to a 1/8-inch circle.
6. Then place another baking sheet on top; this way, the batter is between two baking sheets.
7. Place in an oven and bake for about 8 minutes until the pizza crust is golden brown.
8. For the toppings, place your hamburger in a sauté pan and fry till it's brown, and then wash your mushrooms thoroughly.
9. After the crust is baked, remove the top layer of parchment paper carefully to prevent the froth from sticking to the pizza crust.

10. Put your toppings on top of the crust and bake for an additional 8 minutes.
11. Once ready, slide the pizza off the parchment paper and onto a plate.

Nutrition:

- Calories: 478
- Protein: 30 g
- Carbohydrates: 22 g
- Fats: 29 g

Amaranth Porridge

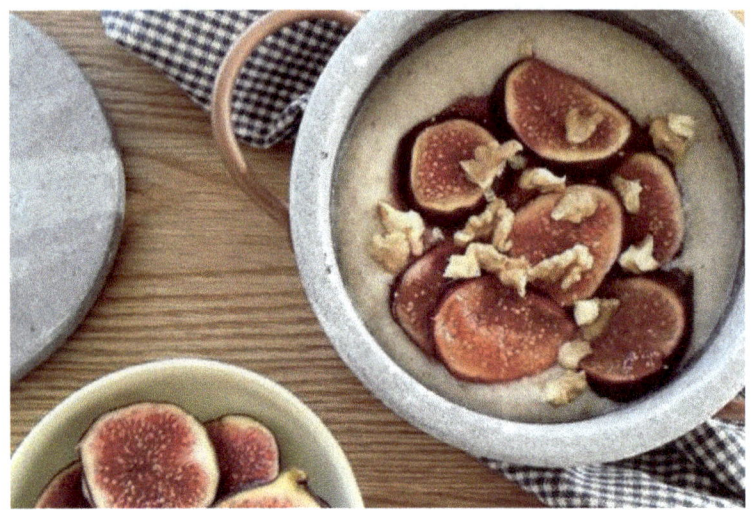

Preparation Time: 5 minutes

Cooking Time: 30 minutes

Servings: 2

Ingredients:

- 2 cups of coconut milk
- 2 cups of alkaline water
- 1 cup of amaranth
- 2 tbsps. Of coconut oil
- 1 tbsp. of ground cinnamon

Directions:

1. In a saucepan, mix in the milk with water, then boil the mixture.
2. Stir in the amaranth, then reduce the heat to medium.
3. Cook on the medium heat, then simmer for a minimum of 30 minutes while stirring occasionally.
4. Turn off the heat.
5. Add in cinnamon and coconut oil then stir.
6. Serve.

Nutrition:

- Calories: 434
- Fat: 35 g
- Carbs: 27 g
- Protein: 6.7 g

Lavender Blueberry Chia Seed Pudding

Preparation Time: 1 hour 10 minutes

Cooking Time: 0 minutes

Servings: 4

Ingredients:

- 100 g of blueberries
- 70 g of organic quark
- 50 g of soy yogurt
- 30 g of hazelnuts
- 200 ml of almond milk
- 2 tbsp. of chia seeds
- 2 teaspoons of agave syrup
- 2 teaspoons of lavender

Directions:

1. Bring the almond milk to a boil alongside the lavender.
2. Let the mixture simmer for 10 minutes at a reduced temperature.
3. Let them calm down afterwards.

4. If the milk is cold, add the blueberries and puree everything.
5. Mix the entire thing with the chia seeds and agave syrup.
6. Let everything soak in the refrigerator for an hour.
7. Mix the yogurt and curd cheese together.
8. Add both to the group.
9. Divide the pudding into glasses.
10. Finely chop the hazelnuts and sprinkle them on top.

Nutrition:

- Kcal: 252
- Carbohydrates: 12 g
- Protein: 1 g
- Fat: 11 g

Coconut Chia Pudding with Berries

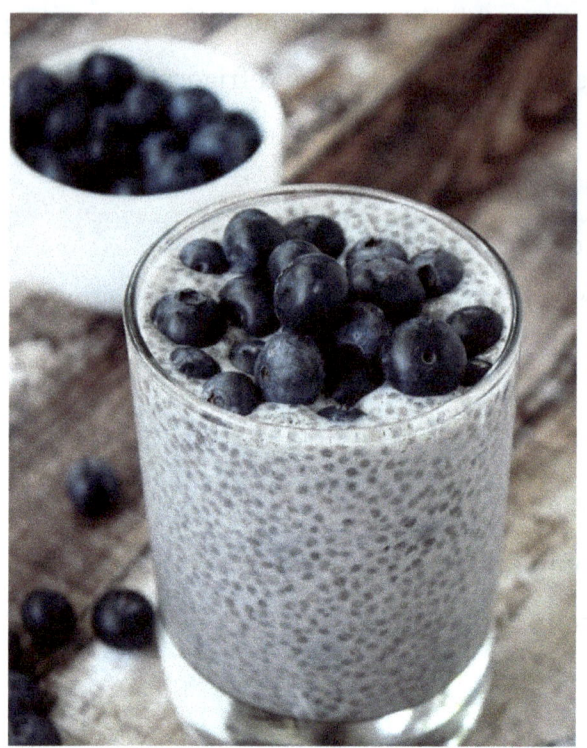

Preparation Time: 20 minutes

Cooking Time: 45 minutes

Servings: 2

Ingredients:

- 150 g of raspberries and blueberries
- 60 g of chia seeds

- 500 ml of coconut milk
- 1 teaspoon of agave syrup
- ½ teaspoon of ground bourbon vanilla

Directions:

1. Put the chia seeds, agave syrup, and vanilla in a bowl.
2. Pour in the coconut milk.
3. Mix thoroughly and let it soak for 30 minutes.
4. Meanwhile, wash the berries and allow them to drain well.
5. Divide the coconut chia pudding between two glasses.
6. Put the berries on top.

Nutrition:

- Kcal: 662
- Carbohydrates: 18 g
- Protein: 8 g
- Fat: 55 g

Omelette with Tomatoes and Spring Onions

Preparation Time: 5 minutes

Cooking Time: 20 minutes

Ingredients:

- 6 eggs
- 2 tomatoes
- 2 spring onions
- 1 shallot
- 2 tbsps. of butter
- 1 tbsp. of olive oil
- 1 pinch of nutmeg salt
- Pepper

Directions:

1. Whisk the eggs in a bowl.
2. Mix them together and season them with salt and pepper.
3. Peel the shallot and chop it up.
4. Clean the onions and cut them into rings.

5. Wash the tomatoes and cut them into pieces.
6. Heat butter and oil in a pan.
7. Braise half the shallots in it.
8. Add half the egg mixture.
9. Let everything set over medium heat.
10. Scatter a couple of tomatoes and onion rings on top.
11. Repeat with the last half of the egg mixture.
12. At the end, spread the grated nutmeg over the entire thing.

Nutrition:

- Kcal: 263
- Carbohydrates: 8 g
- Protein: 20.3 g
- Fat: 24 g

Bacon Cheeseburger

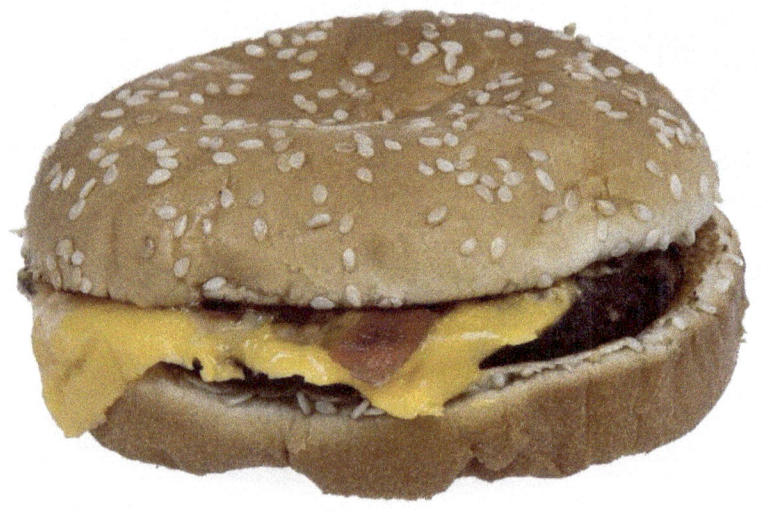

Preparation Time: 5 minutes

Cooking Time: 15 minutes

Servings: 4

Ingredients:

- 1 lb. of lean ground beef
- ¼ cup of chopped yellow onion
- 1 clove of garlic, minced
- 1 tbsp. of yellow mustard
- 1 tbsp. of Worcestershire sauce

- ½ tsp. of salt
- Cooking spray
- 4 ultra-thin slices of cheddar cheese, cut into 6 equal-sized rectangular pieces
- 3 pieces of turkey bacon, each cut into 8 evenly-sized rectangular pieces
- 24 dill pickle chips
- 4-6 green leaf lettuce leaves, torn into 24 small square-shaped pieces
- 12 cherry tomatoes; sliced in half

Directions:

1. Pre-heat oven to 400°F.
2. Combine the garlic, salt, onion, Worcester sauce, and beef in a medium-sized bowl, and blend well.
3. Form mixture into 24 small meatballs. Place meatballs onto a foil-lined baking sheet and cook for 12-15 minutes. Leave oven on.
4. Top every meatball with a bit of cheese, then return to the oven till cheese melts, about 2 to 3 minutes. Let meatballs cool.

5. To assemble bites: on a toothpick, layer a cheese-covered meatball, piece of bacon, piece of lettuce, pickle chip, and a tomato half.

Nutrition:

- Calories: 234
- Protein: 20 g
- Fat: 3 g
- Carbs: 12 g

Chia Seed Gel with Pomegranate and Nuts

Preparation Time: 5 minutes

Cooking Time: 10 minutes

Servings: 3

Ingredients:

- 20 g of hazelnuts
- 20 g of walnuts
- 120 ml of almond milk
- 4 tbsps. of chia seeds
- 4 tbsps. of pomegranate seeds
- 1 teaspoon of agave syrup
- Some lime juices

Directions:

1. Finely chop the nuts.
2. Mix the almond milk with the chia seeds. Let everything soak for 10 to 20 minutes.
3. Occasionally stir the mixture with the chia seeds.

4. Stir in the agave syrup.
5. Pour 2 tablespoons of every mixture into a dessert glass.
6. Layer the chopped nuts on top.
7. Cover the nuts with 1 tablespoon each of the chia mass.
8. Sprinkle the pomegranate seeds on top and serve everything.

Nutrition:

- Kcal: 248
- Carbohydrates: 7 g
- Protein: 1 g
- Fat: 19 g

Pancakes with Berries

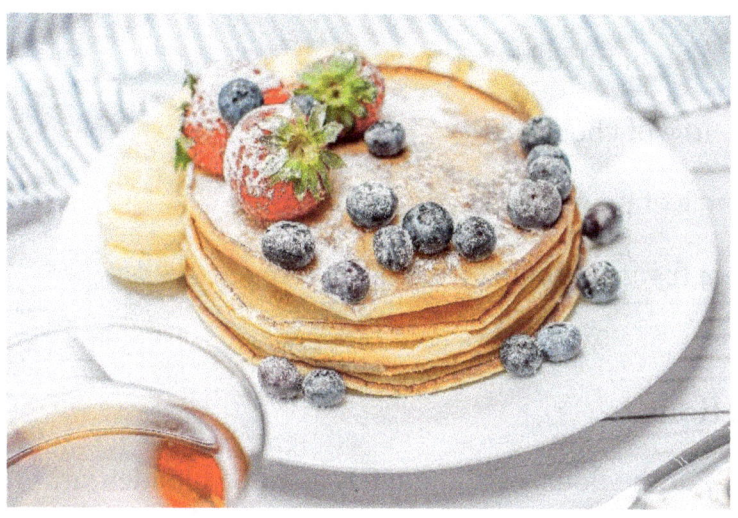

Preparation Time: 5 minutes

Cooking Time: 20 minutes

Servings: 2

Ingredients:

Pancake:

- 1 egg
- 50 g of spelled flour
- 50 g of almond flour
- 15 g of coconut flour

- 150 ml of water salt

Filling:

- 40 g of mixed berries
- 10 g of chocolate
- 5 g of powdered sugar
- 4 tbsps. of yogurt

Directions:

1. Put the flour, egg, and a few salt in a blender jar.
2. Add 150 ml of water.
3. Mix everything with a whisk.
4. Mix everything into a batter.
5. Heat a coated pan.
6. Put in half the batter.
7. Once the pancake is firm, turn it over.
8. Take out the pancake, then add the last half of the batter to the pan and repeat.
9. Melt chocolate over a water bath.
10. Let the pancakes cool.
11. Brush the pancakes with the yogurt.
12. Wash the berry and let it drain.
13. Put berries on the yogurt.
14. Roll up the pancakes.

15. Sprinkle them with the granulated sugar.
16. Decorate the entire thing with the melted chocolate.

Nutrition:

- Kcal: 298
- Carbohydrates: 26 g
- Protein: 21 g
- Fat: 9 g

Porridge with Walnuts

Preparation Time: 5 minutes

Cooking Time: 10 minutes

Servings: 1

Ingredients:

- 50 g of raspberries
- 50 g of blueberries
- 25 g of ground walnuts
- 20 g of crushed flaxseed
- 10 g of oatmeal
- 200 ml of nut drink
- Agave syrup
- ½ teaspoon of cinnamon salt

Directions:

1. Heat the nut drink a little in a saucepan.
2. Add the walnuts, flaxseed, and oatmeal, stirring constantly.
3. Stir in the cinnamon and salt.

4. Simmer for 8 minutes.
5. Keep stirring everything.
6. Sweet the entire mixture.
7. Put the porridge in a bowl.
8. Wash the berries and allow them to drain.
9. Add them to the porridge and serve everything.

Nutrition:

- Kcal: 378
- Carbohydrates: 11 g
- Protein: 18 g
- Fat: 27 g

Omelette à la Margherita

Preparation Time: 10 minutes

Cooking Time: 20 minutes

Servings: 2

Ingredients:

- 3 eggs
- 50 g of parmesan cheese
- 2 tbsps. of heavy cream
- 1 tbsp. of olive oil
- 1 teaspoon of oregano nutmeg
- Salt
- Pepper
- For covering:
- 3-4 stalks of basil
- 1 tomato
- 100 g of grated mozzarella

Directions:

1. Mix the cream and eggs in a medium bowl.
2. Add the grated parmesan, nutmeg, oregano, pepper and salt, and stir everything.
3. Heat the oil in a pan.
4. Add 1/2 of the egg and cream to the pan.
5. Let the omelet set over medium heat, turn it, then remove it.
6. Repeat with the last half of the egg mixture.
7. Cut the tomatoes into slices and place them on top of the omelets.
8. Scatter the mozzarella over the tomatoes.
9. Place the omelets on a baking sheet.
10. Cook at 180 degrees for 5 to 10 minutes.
11. Then take the omelets out and decorate them with the basil leaves.

Nutrition:

- Kcal: 402
- Carbohydrates: 7 g
- Protein: 21 g
- Fat: 34 g

Sweet Cashew Cheese Spread

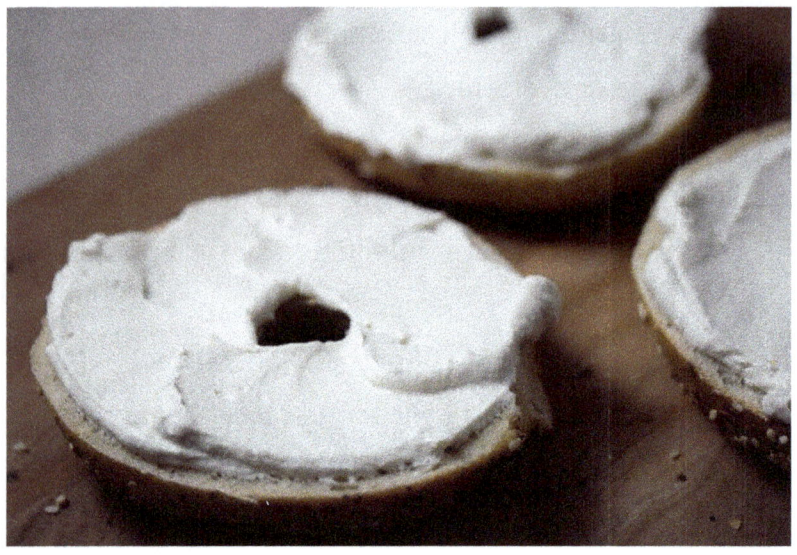

Preparation Time: 5 minutes

Cooking Time: 5 minutes

Servings: 10

Ingredients:

- Stevia (5 drops)
- Cashews (2 cups, raw)
- Water (1/2 cup)

Directions:

1. Soak the cashews in water overnight.
2. Next, drain the surplus water then transfer cashews to a food processor.
3. Add in the stevia and the water.
4. Process until smooth.
5. Serve chilled. Enjoy.

Nutrition:

- Fat: 7 g
- Cholesterol: 0 mg
- Sodium: 12.6 mg
- Carbohydrates: 5.7 g

Personal Biscuit Pizza

Preparation Time: 5 minutes

Cooking Time: 15 minutes

Servings: 1

Ingredients:

- 1 sachet of Lean Select
- Buttermilk Cheddar Herb Biscuit
- 2 tbsp. of cold water
- Cooking spray
- 2 tbsp. of no-sugar-added tomato sauce
- ¼ cup of reduced-fat shredded cheese

Directions:

1. Preheat oven to 350°F.
2. Mix biscuit and water, and spread mixture into a little, circular crust shape onto a greased, foil-lined baking sheet. Bake for 10 minutes.
3. Top with spaghetti sauce and cheese, and cook till cheese is melted, about 5 minutes.

Nutrition:

- Calories: 301
- Protein: 13 g
- Fat: 8
- Carbs: 7

Fried Egg with Bacon

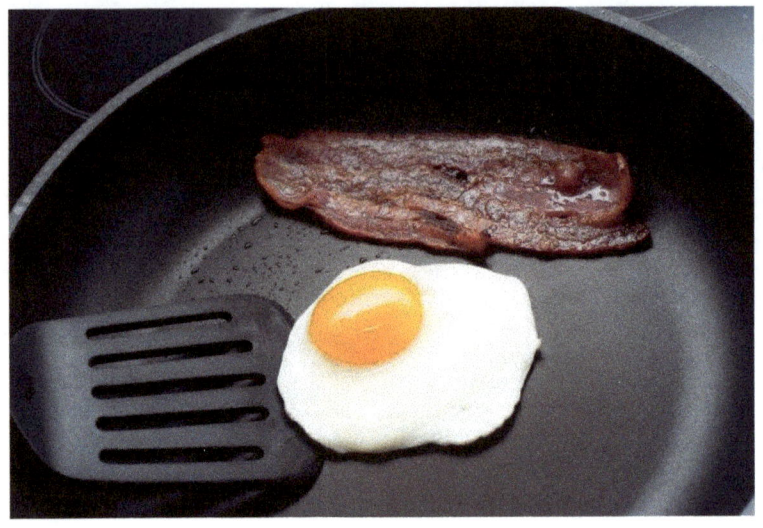

Preparation Time: 5 minutes

Cooking Time: 10 minutes

Servings: 1

Ingredients:

- 2 eggs
- 30 grams of bacon
- 2 tbsps. of olive oil salt
- Pepper

Directions:

1. Heat oil in the pan and fry the bacon.
2. Reduce the heat and beat the eggs in the pan.
3. Cook the eggs and season with salt and pepper.
4. Serve the fried eggs hot with the bacon.

Nutrition:

- Kcal: 405
- Carbohydrates: 1 g
- Protein: 19 g
- Fat: 38 g

Eel on Scrambled Eggs and Bread

Preparation Time: 5 minutes

Cooking Time: 10 minutes

Servings: 2

Ingredients:

- 4 eggs
- 1 shallot
- 4 slices of low carb bread
- 2 sticks of dill
- 200 g of smoked eel
- 1 tbsp. of oil
- Salt
- White pepper

Directions:

1. Mix the eggs in a bowl and season with salt and pepper.
2. Peel the shallot and cut it into fine cubes.
3. Chop the dill.
4. Remove the skin from the eel and cut it into pieces.

5. Heat the oil in a pan and steam the shallot in it.
6. Add in the eggs and allow them to set.
7. Use the spatula to stir the eggs several times.
8. Reduce the heat and add the dill.
9. Stir everything.
10. Spread the scrambled eggs over four slices of bread.
11. Put the eel pieces on top.
12. Add some fresh dill and serve everything.

Nutrition:

- Kcal: 830
- Carbohydrates: 8 g
- Protein: 45 g
- Fat: 64 g

Whole Grain Bread and Avocado

Preparation Time: 5 minutes

Cooking Time: 0 minutes

Serving: 1

Ingredients:

- 2 slices of whole meal bread
- 60 g of cottage cheese
- 1 stick of thyme
- ½ avocado
- ½ lime Chili flakes
- Salt
- Pepper

Directions:

1. Cut the avocado in half.
2. Remove the pulp and cut it into slices.
3. Pour the juice over it.
4. Wash the thyme and shake it dry.
5. Remove the leaves from the stem.

6. Brush the entire wheat bread with the pot cheese.
7. Place the avocado slices on top.
8. Top with the chili flakes and thyme.
9. Add salt and pepper and serve.

Nutrition:

- Kcal: 490
- Carbohydrates: 31 g
- Protein: 19 g
- Fat: 21 g

Cheeseburger Pie

Preparation Time: 25 minutes

Cooking Time: 90 minutes

Servings: 4

Ingredients:

- 1 large spaghetti squash
- 1 lb. of lean ground beef
- ¼ cup of diced onion
- 2 eggs
- 1/3 cup of low-fat, plain Greek yogurt
- 2 Tbsp. of Tomato sauce
- ½ tsp. of Worcestershire sauce
- 2/3 cup of reduced-fat, shredded cheddar cheese
- 2 oz. of dill pickle slices
- Cooking spray

Directions:

1. Preheat oven to 400°F.

2. Slice spaghetti squash in half lengthwise; throw out pulp and seeds. Spray with cooking spray.
3. Place the cut pumpkin halves on a foil-lined baking sheet and bake for 30 minutes. Once cooked, let it cool before scraping the pulp from the squash with a fork to get rid of the spaghetti-like strings. Set aside.
4. Push squash strands in the bottom and up sides of the greased pie pan, creating a good layer.
5. Meanwhile, set up pie filling. In a lightly greased, medium-sized skillet, cook beef and onion over medium heat for 8 to 10 minutes, sometimes stirring, until meat is brown. Drain and take away from heat. Whisk together the eggs, tomato paste, Greek yogurt, Worcester sauce, and add the ground beef mixture. Pour the pie filling over the pumpkin rind.
6. Sprinkle the meat filling with cheese, then fill with pickled cucumber slices.
7. Bake for 40 minutes.

Nutrition:

- Calories: 270
- Protein: 23 g
- Carbohydrate: 10 g
- Fat: 23 g

Asparagus & Crabmeat Frittata

Preparation Time: 5 minutes

Cooking Time: 15 minutes

Servings: 4

Ingredients:

- 2½ tbsp. of extra virgin olive oil
- 2 lbs. of asparagus
- 1 tsp. of salt
- 1 ½ tsp. of black pepper
- 2 tsps. of sweet paprika
- 1 lb. of lump crabmeat
- 1 tbsp. of finely cut chives
- ¼ cup of basil chopped
- 4 cups of liquid egg substitute

Directions:

1. Remove the tough ends of the asparagus and cut it into bite-sized pieces.
2. Preheat an oven to 375°F.

3. In a 12-Inch to a 14-inch oven-proof, non-stick skillet, warm the vegetable oil and boil the asparagus until soft. Season with pepper, paprika, and salt.
4. In a bowl, add the chives, crab and basil meat.
5. Pour in the liquid egg substitute and blend until it has combined.
6. Pour the crab and egg mixture into the skillet with the cooked asparagus and stir to mix. Bake over low to medium heat until the eggs start bubbling.
7. Place the skillet in the oven and bake for about 15-20 minutes until the eggs are golden brown. Serve the dish warm.

Nutrition:

- Calories: 340
- Protein: 50 g
- Carbohydrate: 14 g
- Fat: 10g

Grilled Chicken Power Bowl with Green Goddess Dressing

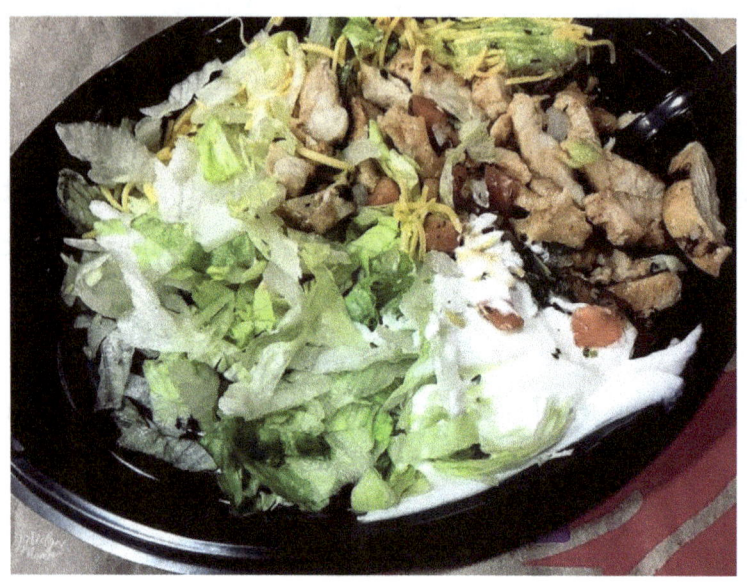

Preparation Time: 5 minutes

Cooking Time: 15 minutes

Servings: 4

Ingredients:

- 1 ½ boneless, skinless chicken breasts
- ¼ tsp. each of salt & pepper
- 1 cup of diced or cubed kabocha squash

- 1 cup of diced zucchini
- 1 cup of diced yellow summer squash
- 1 cup of diced broccoli
- 8 cherry tomatoes, halved
- 4 radishes, sliced thin
- 1 cup of shredded red cabbage
- ¼ cup of hemp or pumpkin seeds

Green Goddess Dressing:

- ½ cup of low-fat plain Greek yogurt
- 1 cup of fresh basil
- 1 clove of garlic
- 4 tbsps. of lemon juice
- ¼ tsp. of each salt & pepper

Directions:
1. Pre-heat oven to 350°F.
2. Season chicken with salt and pepper.
3. Roast chicken for 12 minutes until it reaches a temperature of 165°F. When done, remove from oven and put aside to rest, about 5 minutes. Cut in bite-sized pieces and keep warm.

4. While the chicken rests, steam diced kabocha squash, yellow summer squash, zucchini, and broccoli in a covered microwave-proof bowl for about 5 minutes, till soft.
5. For the dressing, arrange the ingredients in a blender and puree till smooth.
6. To serve, place an equal amount of Veggie Mix into four individual bowls. Add an equal amount of cherry tomatoes, radishes, and chopped cabbage to every bowl alongside 1/4 of the chicken and a tablespoon of seeds.
7. Dress up. Enjoy!

Nutrition:

- Calories: 300
- Protein: 43 g
- Carbohydrate: 12 g
- Fat: 10 g

Yogurt with Granola and Persimmon

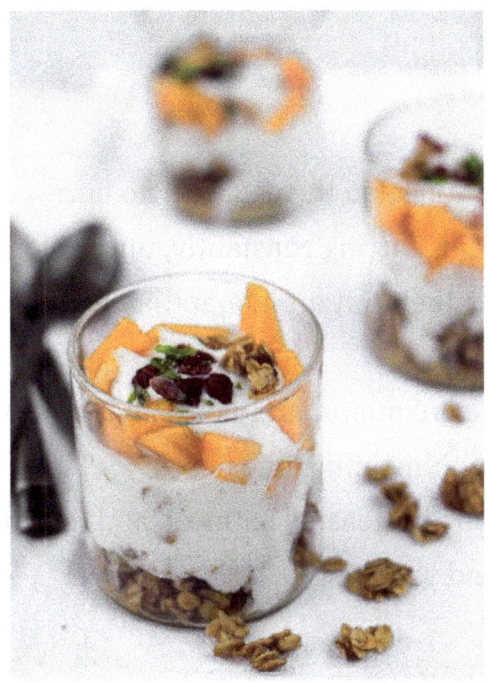

Preparation Time: 5 minutes

Cooking Time: 5 minutes

Servings: 1

Ingredients:

- 150 g of Greek style yogurt
- 20 g of oatmeal

- 60 g of fresh persimmons
- 30 ml of tap water

Directions:

1. Put the oatmeal in the pan with no fat.
2. Toast them, stirring constantly, until golden brown.
3. Then put them on a plate and allow them to cool down briefly.
4. Peel the persimmon and put it in a bowl with the water. Mix everything into a fine puree.
5. Put the yogurt, toasted oatmeal, and the puree in layers in a glass and serve.

Nutrition:

- Kcal: 286
- Carbohydrates: 29 g
- Protein: 1 g
- Fat: 11 g

Smoothie Bowl with Spinach, Mango, and Muesli

Preparation Time: 10 minutes

Cooking Time: 0 minutes

Servings: 1

Ingredients:

150 g of yogurt

30 g of apple

30 g of mango

30 g of low carb muesli

10 g of spinach

10 g of chia seeds

Directions:
1. Soak the spinach leaves and allow them to drain.
2. Peel the mango and cut it into strips.
3. Remove apple core and cut it into pieces.
4. Put everything except the mango alongside the yogurt in a blender and make a fine puree out of them.

5. Put the spinach smoothie in a bowl.
6. Add the muesli, chia seeds, and mango.
7. Serve the whole thing.

Nutrition:

- Kcal: 362
- Carbohydrates: 21 g
- Protein: 12 g
- Fat: 21 g

Smoothie Bowl with Berries, Poppy Seeds, Nuts and Seeds

Preparation Time: 15 minutes

Cooking Time: 0 minutes

Servings: 2

Ingredients:

- 5 chopped almonds
- 2 chopped walnuts
- 1 apple
- ¼ banana
- 300 g of yogurt
- 60 g of raspberries
- 20 g of blueberries
- 20 g of rolled oats; roasted in a pan
- 10 g of poppy seeds
- 1 teaspoon of pumpkin seeds
- Agave syrup

Directions:

1. Clean the fruit and let it drain.
2. Take some berries and set them aside.
3. Place the remaining berries in a tall mixing vessel.
4. Cut the banana into slices, and put a couple of the slices aside.
5. Add the rest of the banana to the berries.
6. Remove the core of the apple and cut it into quarters.
7. Cut the quarters into thin wedges and set a couple of them aside.
8. Add the remaining wedges to the berries.
9. Add the yogurt to the fruits and blend everything into a puree.
10. Sweeten the smoothie with the agave syrup.
11. Divide it into two bowls.
12. Serve it with the remaining fruit, poppy seeds, oatmeal, nuts and seeds.

Nutrition:

- Kcal: 284
- Carbohydrates: 21 g
- Protein: 11 g
- Fat: 19 g

Mini Zucchini Bites

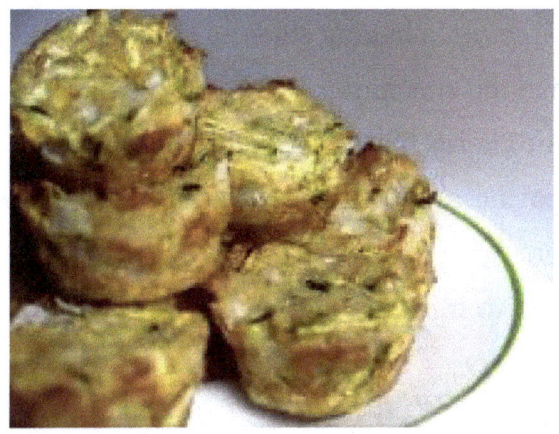

Preparation Time: 10 minutes

Cooking Time: 10 minutes

Servings: 6

Ingredients:

- 1 zucchini, cut into thick circles
- 3 cherry tomatoes; halved
- 1/2 cup of parmesan cheese; grated
- Salt and pepper to taste
- 1 tsp. of chives; chopped

Directions:

1. Preheat the oven to 390º F.
2. Add paper on a baking sheet.
3. Arrange the zucchini pieces.
4. Add the cherry halves on each zucchini slice.
5. Add parmesan cheese, chives, and sprinkle with salt and pepper.
6. Bake for 10 minutes. Serve.

Nutrition:

- Fat: 1.0 g
- Cholesterol: 5.0 mg
- Sodium: 400.3 mg
- Potassium: 50.5 mg
- Carbohydrates: 7.3 g

Beef with Broccoli on Cauliflower Rice

Preparation Time: 5 minutes

Cooking Time: 15 minutes

Servings: 2

Ingredients:

- 1 lb. of raw beef round steak, cut into strips.
- 1 tbsp. + 2 tsp. of low sodium soy sauce
- 1 Splenda packet
- ½ cup of water
- 1 ½ cup of broccoli florets
- 1 tsp. of sesame or olive oil
- 2 cups of cooked, grated cauliflower or frozen diced cauliflower

Directions:

1. Stir steak with soy and allow to sit for about 15 minutes.
2. Heat oil over medium-high heat and fry beef for 3-5 minutes or until browned.
3. Remove from pan.

4. Put broccoli, Splenda, and water in the pan. Cook for 5 minutes or until broccoli starts to appear soft, stirring sometimes.
5. Add beef back in and heat up thoroughly.
6. Serve the dish with cauliflower rice.

Nutrition:

- Calories 201
- Protein: 23 g
- Fat: 4 g
- Carbs: 2 g

Ancho Tilapia on Cauliflower Rice

Preparation Time: 15 minutes

Cooking Time: 30 minutes

Servings: 4

Ingredients:

- 2 lbs. of tilapia
- 1 tsp. of lime juice
- 1 tsp. of salt
- 1 tbsp. of ground ancho pepper
- 1 tsp. of ground cumin
- 1 ½ tbsp. of extra virgin olive oil
- ¼ cup of toasted pumpkin seeds
- 6 cups of cauliflower rice minutes
- 1 cup of coarsely chopped fresh cilantro

Directions:

1. Preheat oven to 450°F.
2. Dress tilapia with juice and put aside.

3. Combine cumin, ancho pepper, and salt in a bowl. Season tilapia with spice mixture.
4. Lay tilapia on a baking sheet or casserole dish and bake for 7 minutes.
5. In the meantime, in a big skillet, boil the cauliflower rice in olive oil till it becomes soft or for about 2-3 minutes.
6. Blend the pumpkin seeds and cilantro into the rice. Remove from heat, and serve.

Nutrition:

- Calories: 350
- Fat: 13 g
- Carbohydrate: 10 g
- Protein: 51 g

Turkey Caprese Meatloaf Cups

Preparation Time: 20 minutes

Cooking Time: 45 minutes

Servings: 6

Ingredients:

- 1 large egg
- 2 pounds of ground turkey breast
- 3 pieces of sun-dried tomatoes, drained and chopped
- ¼ cup of fresh basil leaves, chopped
- 5 ounces of low-fat fresh mozzarella; shredded
- ½ teaspoon of garlic powder
- ¼ teaspoon of salt and ½ teaspoon of pepper, to taste

Directions:

1. Preheat oven to 400°F.
2. Beat the egg in a big bowl.
3. Add the remaining ingredients and blend everything with your hands until they are evenly combined.

4. Spray a 12-cup muffin tin and divide the turkey mixture among the muffin cups, pressing the combination in. Cook in the preheated oven till the turkey is well-cooked or for about 25-30 minutes.
5. Chill the meatloaves entirely and store them in a container in the fridge for up to five days.

Nutrition:

- Calories: 181
- Protein: 43 g
- Fat: 11 g
- Carbs: 9 g

Almond Pancakes

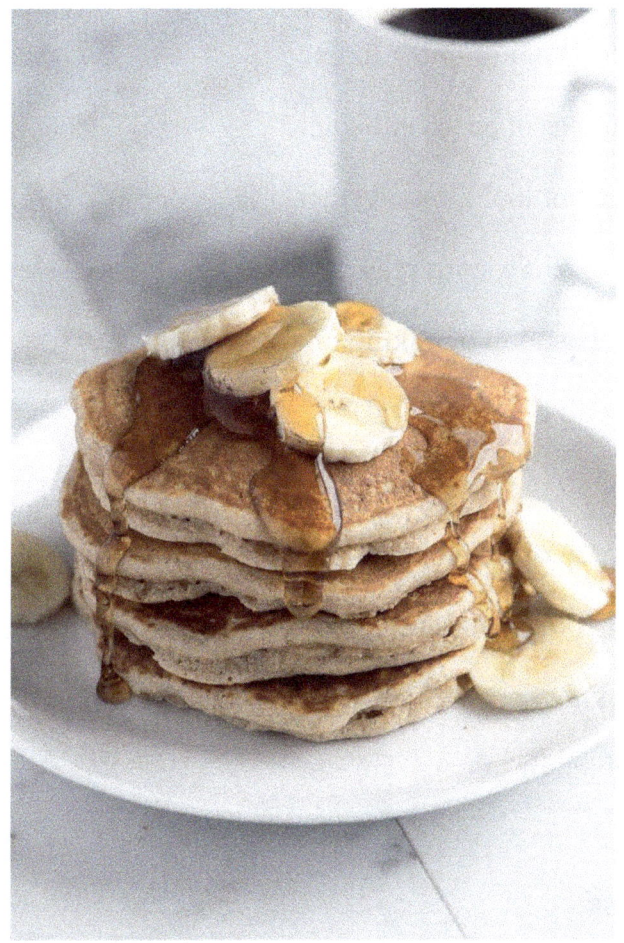

Preparation Time: 10 minutes

Cooking Time: 13 minutes

Servings: 12

Ingredients:

- 6 eggs
- 1/4 cup of almonds; toasted
- 2 ounces of cocoa chocolate
- 1 teaspoon of almond extract
- 1/3 cup of coconut; shredded
- 1/2 teaspoon of baking powder
- 1/4 cup of coconut oil
- 1/2 cup of coconut flour
- 1/4 cup of stevia
- 1 cup of almond milk
- Cooking spray
- A pinch of salt

Directions:

1. Mix coconut flour with stevia, baking powder, salt, coconut, and stir.
2. Add coconut oil, eggs, almond milk and the flavorer and stir well again.
3. Add chocolate and almonds and whisk well again.

4. Heat up a pan and add cooking spray; add 2 tablespoons of batter, spread into a circle, cook until its golden, flip, cook again until it's done and transfer to a pan.
5. Do the same for rest of the batter and serve your pancakes directly.

Nutrition:
- Calories: 266
- Fat: 13 g
- Fiber: 8 g
- Carbs: 10 g
- Protein: 11 g

www.ingramcontent.com/pod-product-compliance
Lightning Source LLC
Chambersburg PA
CBHW071108030426
42336CB00013BA/2000

9781803179070